The Brain a supercomputer and how it affects our physical and emotional wellbeing.

By Maria Sayer

In memory of Mary Margaret McClymont

Contents

Introduction to Trauma

Hello and welcome. How are you doing today? I hope you are doing perfectly well. It is my pleasure to welcome you to our wonderful and unique audiobook on improving the well-being of the human mind and body. I know you have probably already heard other book proposals like the one I am presenting to you, but I ask you to please give us a try, you won't regret it. After all, there is no better way to know if something is genuine or not than to check it out for yourself, or am I wrong?

Well, before I start with the main information of this introduction, I want to say something crucial to you. The information contained here is for your benefit and is based on many studies around the globe. You can search it out if you want to be sure.

Let me ask you the following question, have you ever suffered from any trauma? If you are listening to this, chances are your answer is yes. When you go through a traumatic experience, all that unpleasant information is immediately stored in the supercomputer that is our brain. The human mind is very powerful, capable of doing wonders, but also capable of making us suffer greatly if we do not put a stop to it.

Many times, people who have suffered traumas in their lives tend to have sequels of those experiences. There are cases of adults whose parents yelled at them a lot in their childhood, and even in their adulthood, they cannot stand it when someone raises their

voice too much. When this happens, in their minds, they go back to being those fragile little ones looking for help. They go back to that period of their lives where their trauma originated. That is how powerful the human mind is, but it does not stop there.

I bet you have also heard of the many cases of soldiers and war veterans returning home after many years. Being away for so long, the battlefield becomes their natural habitat; their normality is in the suffering they experience there. The body and mind process all this information and makes these brave soldiers believe that even though they are home, they still feel that they are still in the war.

That is why when they hear a sound as innocent as a balloon popping, a tire bursting, or simply an object falling to the ground, their first instinct is to take refuge, to plant themselves on the ground, to look for a trench, to attack a non-existent enemy, or simply to take shelter just as they would have done on the battlefield. All this is because the supercomputer, which is their mind, has already written a program that was reinforced by their daily routine as soldiers.

Do you understand where I am going with this?

The human brain does not understand which things are real and which are not; it learns by repetition. That is why when we expose it to the same routine repeatedly, it generates in it what we call programs, an action that is engraved in the mind and is executed almost automatically and without less effort.

But what does this have to do with healing trauma and having a healthier life? You may ask. Let me tell you that it has everything to do with it, my friend, we have gotten to the root of the problem.

The real reason why not many people have a full and happy life is simply because they have incorporated junk programs into their minds. In other words, their minds are dominated by negative and self-destructive thoughts that lead them to commit acts that make them unhappy, and thus to lead the life they hate so much.

Can my thoughts influence my life so much? You may ask. The short answer is yes but let me give you an answer that is a little more extensive and backed by science.

There are actual medical records of patients who suffered from both mild and terminal illnesses. In both cases, the patients were given the same treatments, and there was no variation in the amount or severity of illness. And yet, one group of those patients was more likely to be cured of their disease, while others were much slower to heal, stayed as they were, or just did not make it at all.

Believe it or not, what primarily helped the healthy patients in their recovery was a simple but powerful change of mindset. Positive thinking helps more than you think, and quantum physics supports this idea.

Dr. Masaru Emoto was responsible for leading amazing research in which he demonstrated that, depending on our positive or negative mood, we can change the structure of water molecules. It sounds like science fiction, but it is pure quantum physics.

But not only can we change the water molecules depending on our mood, but we can also change or heal our own. Terminally ill patients, people with depression and attachment problems, people with severe childhood trauma, or simply someone who is somewhat depressed, I come to you to tell you that a change of focus can powerfully put you back in control of your life.

We will accomplish this by implementing positive self-talk, along with some meditation exercises, conscious breathing, physical exercise, etc.

If our mind is a computer, and so far, the program that has been running in it has done nothing but bring us pure misfortune, well my friend, it is time to uninstall it and replace it with a better and healthier one.

We have the power to heal ourselves. So come, give me your hand; it is time to start healing.

Relax Mind and Body

Greetings, how are you feeling? I hope you are perfectly well and healthy. It is an honor and a great joy for me to have you here with me, in this new guided meditation. This will be step number one on the road to your recovery and the first step to becoming that wonderful person you know you are inside but has not yet fully emerged.

Remember, the first step can always be the hardest but do not be afraid, remember that you are not alone in this. Remember, I will be always here with you, guiding you with my voice, so there is nothing to fear.

Very well, the first step on the way to our well-being is to know how to relax both our mind and our body. That is right, in this opportunity, we will practice calmness, using meditation for this purpose.

If you have never meditated in your life, do not worry, I will guide you; you just have to trust me. So, relax, put on a big smile, and embrace the experience. Are you ready? All right, let us get started.

Start by finding a place where you feel comfortable to sit and meditate. It can be anywhere like your bedroom, your living room or your beautiful garden, the important thing is that you feel comfortable in it. Also, make sure that it is free from noises and that it is at a time of the day when no one will disturb you. We do not want distractions. I will give you a moment to find this place; take your time.

Now that you are in your meditation space, find a comfortable place to sit. It can be a chair, a couch, an armchair, a mat on the floor, or even your bed. The key is to feel comfortable and safe.

Once you find it, proceed to sit upright in the place, with your back always straight, but without generating tension or discomfort. Let your hands fall in your lap, let your legs fall on the floor, or you can also cross them as if you were doing yoga, as you prefer. Relax your face, let your shoulders and head fall under their own weight, relax your abdominal area and back, and let your body simply release any tension that ails it at that moment.

Good, you are doing great.

Now that you have a relaxed posture, it is time to gently close your eyes, and begin to breathe in a very slow and deep way. The type of breathing that we will use for these meditation sessions is a very well-known one in this field. It is called diaphragmatic breathing or breathing with the abdomen.

It consists of the following, every time you take a breath through your nose, instead of taking the oxygen to your chest as you normally do, take it to your abdomen, and then exhale through your mouth normally.

Go ahead and try it; you know what to do. I will give you a few minutes to get used to how to breathe this way.

Okay, that is it, you are getting the idea. Very well done. Inhale through your nose, bring the oxygen up to your abdomen, fill it as full as you can with air, and then exhale through your mouth gently open, feeling the body empty of air.

And that is it, see how simple it is? But it does not end here; there is still the most important thing to do. To ensure a state of absolute relaxation to both our mind and our body, it is not enough to inhale and exhale air. We must also feel every part of the process of that inhalation and exhalation.

The temperature, the rhythm, the tingling in our lips, the feeling of relaxation in our muscles, all that we should feel while we breathe. Normally you do not pay attention to the way you breathe, but today you will, and I know you will do great. You can do it, focus. Ready? Here we go.

Inhale now, fill your abdomen with air. Feel the oxygen pass through your nostrils, feel it travel all the way up to your lungs, and feel, as you inhale, how it widens your stomach more and more as you inhale.

And now exhale, feeling the same path, but in reverse, feel how the air now comes out warmly from your mouth and lips. Take a moment to rest at the end of each breath.

Rest in stillness. That is, become fully aware of this present moment; nothing else matters. It is natural if distracting thoughts appear in your mind. You simply refocus your attention on your breath, it is that simple.

Inhale deeply, and then exhale. You are doing great; I will leave you alone for a few minutes to continue your own. I will be right back.

How does your body feel? Doesn't it feel great? I can bet it does. Conscious breathing has helped to slowly relax all your thoughts, and at the same time, by having our mind occupied with how we breathe, we do not leave time for negative thoughts to tense our body.

Breathing and relaxing sounds simple, but sometimes the simplest thing can be the most powerful. Always keep this in mind when meditating.

Okay, it is time to return to the awareness of the physical world, so concentrate on your breathing as much as you can as you have been doing so far. When you are ready, you can open your eyes very slowly, but do not move too fast. Stretch and feel every part of your body right where you are sitting.

Congratulations, you have just successfully completed this session, I congratulate you. See you next time, see you later.

Body Scan

Nice to see you again. How are you feeling today? I hope you are doing great. What a pleasure it is for me to welcome you here with me once again in this new guided meditation that will help you improve your quality of life. You took the first step in your recovery with our previous meditation; let me congratulate you for that. Not many dares to start something new, much less a change as big as the one you have proposed.

Even so, only the first step is not enough. There are still many other steps to take along the way. This will be your second step in this journey of recovery. In it, we will focus on scanning and healing each part of our beloved body.

As we previously decided to relax and let go of tensions, that generated in our body an abrupt change, as it is normally used to negative energy and always being stressed. We sow what we reap, and in this opportunity, we will perceive the fruits of a relaxed and peaceful body.

Remember that there is nothing to fear at all; you are not alone. I will always be here with you, guiding you with my voice, so there is nothing to worry about. You just start to relax and let yourself be carried away by the wonderful experience.

Are you ready? Perfect, let us get started then.

Start by finding a comfortable place to start meditating, it can be anywhere you want. It can be your bedroom, the living room of your home, a study, or even your backyard. If you have a beautiful garden full of many plants like me, I recommend you do it there, you will see that it is a beautiful experience.

I will leave you a moment to choose this place, there is no rush. You can choose calmly.

Well, now that you have an ideal space to meditate, it is time to choose a comfortable place to sit. You can use a chair, a piece of furniture, a sofa, or even a yoga mat, the important thing is that you feel comfortable.

Choose your ideal spot, I will give you a moment.

Perfect, now I want you to sit, and keep your back always straight, but not too much, the idea is not to generate discomfort, just to have a good posture. If you feel extremely uncomfortable, you can put a cushion behind your lower back; there is no problem with doing that.

You can interlace your hands or let your arms rest on your lap. Release your legs and thighs, relax your abdominal area and back, let the weight of your shoulders and head relax back on themselves, relax your abdominal area, and back, and most importantly, please let go of that frown. Your facial muscles will thank you immensely, trust me.

Your posture is now ideal to start meditating. Congratulations.

Now, I will ask you to gently close your eyes and begin to breathe slowly and deeply. Remember to take all the oxygen to the area of your abdomen, to the center of your body. That is it, let's start.

Inhale, fill your abdomen completely with air...and exhale, feeling how your body becomes heavy and how the air caresses the inside of your cheeks and lips. Today I want you to focus on each of your breathing sensations. It will be extremely helpful for what comes next.

You just breathe. I will be back with you in a few moments. Just look, you have become fully conscious of your breathing, but what great happiness.

Perfect then, we will start the body scan of your body. How do we do that? Simple, just as the name implies, it will be as if we pass a giant scanner that will be in charge of inspecting that our whole body is fine. When I name a part of your body, you will bring your attention to it and verify that everything is in order. It is as simple as that. Ready? Here we go.

Breathe, breathe calmly, I want you to bring your attention to the soles of your feet, feel this area. Give yourself a few minutes to feel the ground you are walking on at this very moment. What temperature is it? Is it warm? Is it cold? Feel it in detail.

Now go up, and focus your attention on your toes, you can move them if you want. Move them, feel them, they are many toes, verify that each one of them can move correctly and without problems.

We go up a little more, and you get to the part of the tibiae and the calves. These are already a bit bigger muscles, so you will have to pay special attention to them. Feel these muscles. Are they stiff, are they relaxed? Describe every sensation that comes to your mind.

Continuing upwards. We are now in the pelvic area. This area connects with your thighs and buttocks and the beginning of your abdomen. Feel all this area, try to relax it as much as possible; it is not a place that you want to be in tension.

We continue up until we reach the trunk; this large area encompasses the area of your abdomen and your back. When we sit, we tend to tense our abdomen a little bit, and when we have a bad posture, we damage our lower back. I want you to relax these areas and make them feel extremely comfortable.

We go up a little bit more until we get to the chest, shoulders, and neck area. Release the tension; they are not carrying any weight right now, so you do not need to squeeze them or work them. Just release them from that tension that has been bothering them so much. Relax your arms, wrist, and hands, feel any tension and let it go.

We have reached the top, the human head. I want you to feel your face and stop forcing any facial expression. Do not frown, let your tongue relax, do not wrinkle your face; relax it completely. Try to feel how your whole face relaxes, your jaw leaves any tension, and you feel a deep relaxation that you have never felt before.

Good, you have done wonderfully. I congratulate you enormously for that. You can now open your eyes; the body scan is finished. You are healthy and very relaxed. You feel that peace caresses every corner of your body and your being. That is all, see you soon, my dear friend.

Your Inner Self

Greetings, how are you feeling on this beautiful day? I hope you are very well. I warmly welcome you to this new journey. It is my pleasure to be your guiding voice again through this meditation to improve our mental and physical well-being.

Before I begin, I want to offer you my sincere congratulations. Not everyone gets as far as you have come and even less for such a noble goal as the one you have set for yourself. What goal am I talking about? Well, personal improvement, of course.

Most people simply ignore their problems and live with that regret for the rest of their lives, but not you, do you hear me? You are not one of them; today, you have decided to move forward on your path to be a better person who speaks very well of how amazing you already are. No joke, you are admirable.

And speaking of who you really are, that is what our meditation today focuses on. You may have doubted or been made to doubt many times about what kind of person you are or what your likes, times, or goals should be. But, this time, you will connect with your inner self, embrace it, and accept it into your heart.

There is no need to pretend to be someone else; the person you already are wonderful!

Remember well, there is nothing to be afraid of here. I will always be guiding you with my voice through this experience, so you can rest easy. You just relax and let yourself go through the experience. Are you ready? Perfect then, let us get started.

As a first step, find a pleasant place where you can meditate at ease. Your bedroom could be a good place, or even a study, if you do not already have your own meditation room. Remember to do this at a time of the day when you are not working and when you know that no one will disturb you.

I will give you a few minutes to find this place and come back when you are in it.

Perfect, now that we have found our harmonious space, we will proceed to sit on a comfortable surface. It could be a chair or an armchair, even your bed will do, or if you are a bit more rustic, you could even sit on the floor. Everything is up to you.

Settle down; I will give you a few minutes. Keep your back always straight, but not excessively, so that at no time do you feel that you are forcing the posture of your back.   Let your hands fall on your lap, let your feet rest comfortably on the floor without pushing them, relax your shoulders and neck, and let your head fall on its own weight.

Get used to this posture; get used to having no tension in your body.

Now please, I ask you to close your eyes and begin to breathe in a slow and very deep way, concentrating totally on every little aspect of your breathing. Remember, the protagonist of our breathing will be the abdomen, it will help us flow the sensations of relaxation.

Okay, concentrate on your breathing. Inhale, inhale as deeply as possible…and now exhale, feeling how the abdomen becomes small and how your whole body is emptied of oxygen. It is not necessary to immediately restart the breath; just take a short break at the end of each one. Rest in the stillness and silence of this present moment.

You are doing very well; keep it up. Inhale, feel the passage of oxygen from your nose into your lungs, and exhale, resting briefly at the end of the breathing cycle.

Give yourself a little moment to feel your body; it is more relaxed, isn't it? Yes, it is.

I will leave you for a few minutes while you continue to breathe consciously. I will be right back.

Well, what do you know, you have managed to become one with your breathing, congratulations? Our body breathes, and we just pay attention to it, that is all.

Well, let us change the subject of all that a little bit. It is time to finally connect with that inner self, the one that you can sometimes hide from others out of fear or embarrassment. I want you to understand that doing that is perfectly natural; no one likes to get hurt, let alone be criticized. However, being ourselves should not embarrass us. On the contrary, it should be our reason to smile.

I want you to imagine with me the following scenario, try to visualize it as rich in detail as you can. You are a young child, and you are in school. A traumatic place for many, maybe for you too.

There is a group of children gathered talking about things they like, like their favourite TV shows or other things. You approach very confidently and friendly to share your likes and dislikes. However, you are not well received. The children make fun of you, and you walk away very embarrassed.

I know, I know, it is not the picture of hope you were hoping for, but do not lose hopes up. It is not over yet.

Despite being hurt, you see another group of children again talking about the things that make them happy. You decide to be brave and open your heart to them again. This time the result is different. They accept you, or maybe not only that, but they are also completely happy to have someone like you join them, as they consider you unique and wonderful. Much better, isn't it?

Think about the person you are, the things you like, your hobbies, plans, dreams, and friends, and be proud of everything that makes you who you are. You may have debated at some point whether it was wrong to be the way you are, but I say to you, being who you are will always be okay.

Smile, you have managed to accept yourself without a filter. Bravo. Slowly open your eyes and stretch your body. You have successfully completed this session. See you, take care of yourself.

You Are Valuable

It is nice to see you again. How are you feeling today? I hope you are very well and in excellent health, both physically and mentally. It is my pleasure to welcome you back to this safe space for another guided meditation. It never bores me to greet you; I hope it happens often.

This time, I bring you a meditation a little different from the others. If you are one of those people who do not like sudden changes, do not worry. Seriously, there is nothing wrong; we will just incorporate a new and wonderful theme this time.

And what will that theme be? You may ask. Well, that theme is yourself. Yes, as you heard, today we will focus on highlighting all those characteristics that make you such a great and amazing person so that you can keep it always at the forefront of your brain.

We often see people with great talents, jobs, or skills, and when we see them, the first thing we think is, "Wow, they are so amazing, I bet they don't have a single ounce of insecurity in their bodies. I wish I were like them." That is a general thought. But surprise, surprise, things are never that simple.

Even sports pros and movie stars have insecurities, which are fed daily because they are extremely exposed to the public eye. That is right, even those who are beautiful and talented have it a little tough. But, if that is the case, how do they overcome all their problems? You may ask. The answer is simple, they simply must remember that they are valuable people.

In the case of celebrities, they have thousands of fans who constantly flatter them and remind them of how amazing they are. In the case of most people, there are always family and friends who remind you that you are someone great.

We will connect with all your virtues and remind you of the immense value you have as a person.

Do not be afraid; remember that I will always be here for you, helping you with our journey. You just have to relax and let yourself be carried away by this wonderful experience. Are you ready? Perfect then, let us get started.

First, you must find a peaceful place where you can meditate without distractions. I would recommend your bedroom or any other place where you feel comfortable; it is entirely up to you where you feel at peace.

Go on, find this place. I will wait for you in the meantime.

Once we have our practice space, we will proceed to sit on a comfortable surface. It can be a chair, a sofa, or an armchair; even a yoga mat on the floor will do if you are comfortable. Settle in; I will give you a few moments alone to finish.

Okay, now let us work a little on that posture. The recommended posture for meditation is with your back straight but never tense. Let your hands rest on your lap, relax your legs and let your feet drop to the floor; relax your midriff, and let your shoulders and neck drop along with the weight of your head.

Let go of all your tensions. You do not need them where we are going. Congratulations, now you have the right posture to start the practice.

Close your eyes and begin to breathe diaphragmatically, that is, taking all the oxygen from your nose to the area of your abdomen. By breathing in this way, the oxygen is absorbed in a better way by our body, we improve the blood flow, and therefore also help the relaxation of our muscles.

Come on, I want you to practice with me to concentrate and breathe consciously.

Inhale now, fill your abdomen with fresh air, feel it expand as much as it can.... and then exhale, letting the air out gently through your slightly open mouth. Just relax and breathe while being aware of the great blessing of being alive, of the sacred gift of breathing.

I want you to practice it on your own until you have become one with your breath. I will leave you alone for a few minutes. I will be right back. I see with pride that you have managed to focus your mind totally on the breath. Very well done.

Now it is time to connect with those beautiful feelings for you. It is time for you to finally realize once and for all how valuable you really are.

Look at you; someone has congratulated you for the excellent work you have done this week. Inside you tell yourself that it was no big deal, but no, if they congratulate you, it is for something. Do not minimise what you worked so hard for. You are worthy of the recognition you have just received.

How many times have you had a beautiful gesture with someone you love very much? If you want to think about it a little bit, I bet there were many more than you remember. There it is only a truly wonderful person like you is capable of such acts of generosity towards others.

You are worthy, you are beautiful, you are wonderful, and you are someone very valuable. If, at some point, your mind starts trying to convince you otherwise, then change that corrupt program, and replace it with all those times that someone else knew how to recognize your true value.

Learn to take care of your needs, to give yourself the loving space you deserve. A good exercise is to start focusing on dedicating some time for yourself, not only for others. Remember that if you do not listen to yourself, no one will listen to you. Start prioritizing your needs, what you like, what you want. All this has nothing to do with selfishness; it is how to love yourself more and be happy.

You are worth a lot, always keep that in mind. But do not be afraid, I can also remind you whenever you need it. Well, now you can open your eyes and stretch your body. We have successfully completed this session. Remember to smile and remember that you are sensational. See you next time.

Work with Your Cells using quantum physics

Hello, dear friend. How are you feeling today? I hope you are doing great. It is wonderful for me to have you back on this journey. Today I bring you a new guided meditation, which will help you on your way to better mental and physical health.

Before we begin, I want to ask you a little question, do you know about quantum physics and the study of cells? If your answer is yes, you are probably familiar with the magnificent work of Dr. Masaru Emoto. If you say no, do not worry, we are going to learn a little about his research.

Dr. Masaru conducted groundbreaking research, in which he demonstrated that we could change the structure of water molecules through our thoughts and moods. But not only the water molecules but it was also shown that we can directly influence to transform our own cells, this has been researched by many scientists.

Whether you have been suffering from a serious illness for some time, or you have a physical injury that you would like to heal faster, or you have some childhood trauma or sadness, the power of positive self-talk and change in our cells is something so beneficial that it may sound unreal at times. But we believe in evidence here, so it is time to put this great power into practice.

That is right, Today, we will work with your cells so that you can finally heal all that you so desperately need.

Remember, there is nothing to fear during this journey, as I will always be with you, accompanying you with my voice. It is always good to have a friend for the important things, and you have me, so you can rest assured.

You just let yourself go and embrace the experience. Are you ready? All right then, let us get started.

Start by finding a peaceful place where you can meditate at ease, preferably at a time of day when you know no one is going to call you or disturb you in any way. You can settle in your room, in your living room, or even on your terrace. It would be fantastic to have a place full of plants where you can settle in; they always give great natural energy.

I will give you a moment to find your place. I will be right back.

Once you have found your practice space, proceed to sit on a comfortable surface. You cannot practice lying down, as you run the risk of falling asleep in the middle of the session. Likewise, your bed could be a comfortable place to sit, or perhaps a cushioned chair you have lying around, whichever you like best. Find your seat and settle in peacefully. I will give you a moment.

Now let us correct that posture of yours; the recommended posture is with your back always straight, but never tense, perfectly aligned with gravity. If this causes you discomfort, you can also lean your back against the back of the chair, there is no problem with that.

Drop your hands in your lap, relax your legs and feet, relax your shoulders, your neck, your abdomen, your jaw, your head, and relax all your facial muscles and relax your tongue, we do not want any frowns interfering with our relaxation.

Now you can gently close your eyes and begin to breathe in a calm and very deep way using your abdomen. Remember, while breathing, pay full attention to every detail of the breath; nothing else matters.

Inhale now, fill your abdomen with pure air...and exhale, feeling your body empty of air little by little, without tension, without expectation, without effort. Give yourself permission to rest at the end of each breath, rest in the silence of the present moment. That way, you are doing it very well.

It does not matter if at some point, your mind gets distracted; that is completely natural. If it happens to you, simply refocus your attention on the breath; it is as simple as that.

Inhale deeply at this moment...and now exhale, feeling the oxygen travel through your whole body.

I will leave you for a few moments. Do not be worried. I will be back in a few minutes; you just keep going as you are.

Okay, now we will focus on working our cells and healing them little by little. But how to do this? You may ask, well, I am telling you, it is simple. To achieve this, we will use visualization and positive talk.

I want you to imagine all the cells inside your body; they are an infinity, which is true, but I want you to concentrate on a specific one. Go ahead and try it.

What does this cell sound like? Does it have a particular sound? It is said that a healthy cell has a high-pitched sound, and a distressed cell has a rather distorted sound. If your cell has a distorted sound, then we will send positive healing to it.

Go ahead, visualize that high-pitched sound you would like the cell to make, and start saying nice, positive things aloud to it so that it will listen to you and want to heal. A cell is like a plant; kind words help it to heal. Do not be afraid, believe in this, and say the first thing that comes to your mind.

How does this cell sound now? Does it have a higher pitched sound? Well, congratulations, you have done it. You have healed one of the many cells in your body. Now let us go for something much bigger.

Focus on your cells again, but not on one, but a much larger set of them. Concentrate on their sound, that distorted sound which tells you that something is wrong. Now breathe and begin to generate positive thoughts and words that help in its healing. That is it, just like that. You are doing great. Remember you can focus on a particular part of your body each you use this script.

Congratulations, you have succeeded in changing the flow of your cells. They now have a very healthy, high-pitched sound, and your body now feels great, doesn't it?

Well, you can open your eyes now; we are done for this session. See you next time.

Reprogramming Your Supercomputer (brain)

Nice to see you again. How are you feeling today? I hope you are doing great. I am truly happy that once again, I can join you in this wonderful new guided meditation.

In this opportunity, I bring for you a meditation, in which we will take care of replacing that black cloud that you have always carried over you for a vast, healing, and wonderful clear sky. That is right, my friend, it is time to call the technician because we are going to replace those corrupted files that do so much damage to the supercomputer that is your mind.

How is this accomplished? You may ask, it is much simpler than you think. Our brain learns through repetition, if you tell someone enough times that they are stupid over time, they will believe it. Maybe many people doubted you in the past and insulted you, and that is why today you have sad and destructive thoughts.

But do not be alarmed; everything has a solution. Now that we know that the key is repetition, we will simply start running a new and much friendlier program in your mind, repeating, and highlighting each of your amazing qualities until there is no trace left of your former fears.

Remember, the key is repetition. If you tell yourself something enough times and believe it, it will come true, no matter what it is.

Fear not, I will always be with you throughout this experience, accompanying you with my voice, as your friend that I am. You just have to relax and let yourself be carried away by the experience. Are you ready? Very well, let us start then.

Start by finding a comfortable place to start meditating. It can be anywhere you want. You can do it in your bedroom, your living room, look, even your bathroom is a valid option if you feel comfortable there, but take care that no one enters and distract you.

I will give you a few moments to choose this place carefully.

Well, now that you have it, proceed to sit on a comfortable surface. You can use your favorite chair or even sit on your bed. If you are someone a little more rustic, the floor is also an option; as long as you feel comfortable, I recommend using a mat, so you do not hurt your lower back. Come on, settle in. I will give you a moment.

Time to correct that misaligned posture you might have. Place your back always straight, but without putting any pressure on it. We do not want to feel uncomfortable at any time. You can lean your back against the back of your chair if you feel uncomfortable; there is no problem with that.

Relax your legs and let your feet fall comfortably on the floor, relax your arms, let your shoulders, neck, and head fall under their own weight, loosen the muscles of your face, and make sure not to tense your back. Well, that pose is already taking shape. That is great!

Close your eyes very gently, and please begin to breathe in a slow and very deep way, as deep as you can. Remember to bring all the oxygen from your nose to your abdominal area; diaphragmatic breathing is the most useful for this type of meditation.

That is it. Inhale now, fill your abdomen with air...and exhale, feeling the air travel out of your abdomen.

Let us go again. Inhale, fill your abdomen with air, feel your whole belly widen as you inhale and hold...and now exhale, feeling the relaxation of your belly and all your muscles as you expel the oxygen from your body.

Remember that it is not enough just to breathe. You must also pay attention to the way you breathe. If we concentrate on breathing, then there will be no room in our minds for our fears and insecurities; that is the trick of it all.

You cannot see what you do not pay attention to. Always remember that. Keep breathing with the same rhythm as before, do not try to change it for anything in the world, just let it follow its natural flow. Our body breathes on its own, and we only pay attention to it; it is as easy as that. I will leave you a few minutes to enjoy your breathing; I will be right back.

Well, it is finally time to do what we came for. That is right, we are going to replace right now that corrupted file in your brain full of negativity with a kinder and more hopeful one.

Now please listen. I want you to imagine a park or someplace like this. I want you now to recall an experience you have had in that place. Since you still have a corrupted file in your brain, chances are that a bad memory has come to mind.

Negative things happen and cannot be erased. But that does not mean you have to keep reminding yourself of them. Imagine that same park or place but try to remember something good that happened to you there this time. It does not matter how small it was if it was happy.

There it is, you, see? There is no need to bring to your mind a bad memory when you have a much happier one stored in your mind. Now every time you remember this place, I want you to focus on the positive feelings and emotions that happened there.

Focus on your happiness, laughter, smile, the time you spent with others, and anything that makes you feel warm in your chest. Good, you are doing great.

Now, I want you to remember those feelings of happiness and multiply them more and more in your consciousness. It does not matter if only one happy memory comes to mind or a few. Focus on the feelings of joy they make you feel.

The key is repetition, so leave behind that habit of thinking about depressing things and replace it with memories or fantasies that make you happy.

Keep at it, be happy in your mind. Once you are happy there, you will be able to manifest that happiness to the entire world.

Well, now you can open your eyes and stretch your whole body little by little. Congratulations, you have successfully reprogrammed your mind. Congratulations. See you next time.

Just Believe in Yourself

Hello and welcome once again; how are you feeling on this wonderful new day? I hope you are very well and fully healthy, health is always the most important thing. For my part am incredibly happy, as we can be together again, sharing a new guided meditation.

This meditation is quite different from the others because we will deal with a very particular and unexplored topic. Can you guess what it is? I will give you a hint, that subject is you. That is right, in this opportunity, we will focus on igniting your faith in yourself and in everything you have learned so far.

I think I have already told you this once, but please allow me to repeat it. If at some point you come to think that all this is useless, then let me tell you one thing, you will be right. But, on the contrary, if you really have genuine faith in yourself and in everything you have worked for so far, then you will be able to reap the sweet fruits of happiness and your efforts.

It may sound crazy, but it is faith that really makes things happen. If you plant a tree and give it the best possible care but still have no faith in it to grow, then its chances of being born are abysmally diminished.

It may sound cheesy, but if you really want results, then you must believe that they are possible to achieve. Remember how powerful the mind is. It is in charge of making everything we think come true, whether it is positive or negative. So, better to think positively, don't you think so? Well, you get the idea.

Remember that there is nothing to be nervous about; I will always be with you, guiding you with my soft voice, so you can walk calmly. You just relax and let yourself be carried away by the experience. Are you ready? Very well, let us begin.

Start by finding a comfortable place where you can meditate without interruptions. Your bedroom is always a viable choice, maybe even your living room, terrace, or even the guest room. Any place that inspires peace serves the purpose. I will give you a moment to choose this place. No rush, take your time.

Once you have found your ideal spot, it will be time to sit on a comfortable surface. You can choose a chair, a couch, or an armchair. The bed itself is also a viable option if you are not going to fall asleep. I will give you a moment to choose; comfort takes time, after all.

Time to focus on our posture. Start by positioning your back straight, aligned with gravity, but without putting too much force or pressure on it. Remember, the point of all this is for you to be comfortable, so adjust your back posture as you like it.

Relax your arms and let them fall quietly into your lap, release your legs, and let them rest comfortably on the floor, relieve the pressure on your back and abdomen, release the tension in your shoulders and neck, and let your head and facial muscles relax a little at a time. That is it; that pose has already taken the desired shape, very well done.

Now, close your eyes and start to breathe diaphragmatically, slowly, and as deeply as possible. Remember that it is not only and exclusively about breathing. You must also pay special attention to the way you breathe.

Only in this way is it possible to enter the awareness of the present moment. Go ahead and try it. Inhale right now, fill your belly with air... and exhale, feeling the warm air gently touching your lips. Rest at the end of each breath, in stillness, in silence, in calm. If at any moment you feel that your breathing is not deep enough, then do not try to change it. Just let it be it is perfect as it is.

That is, breathe this present moment. This moment lacks nothing, has nothing left over, is completely perfect, and is perfect just as it is.

Now, it is time to change the theme of this meditation a little bit, but still, keep breathing as you have been doing so far. Get ready, for we will connect with your feelings of faith in yourself and all that you have learned so far.

Let me ask you a question, have you felt any significant change since you started these meditation sessions? I do not think you would have made it this far otherwise, so I assume your answer is more than positive.

It seems crazy how something as simple as positive thinking can influence our lives so much, but you have seen the results firsthand. And no, it was not luck or mere coincidence; this whole new being that you are now has been formed because you believed blindly in the process and yourself.

I think we have hit on the keyword belief. While this is not exactly something that is highly recommended to do in every aspect of your life, holding something you do well in high esteem indeed increases your chances of success.

Just look at yourself; you are a completely different being than when you started. Maybe your corrupted files are not healed yet, but you are still much better than when you started with this program.

You have done very well, but that is no reason to stop here. On the contrary, you must continue to apply what you have learned in your day-to-day life. Live, be happy, think positive every chance you get, and you will see how the rewards of the world will fall upon you.

You have done a great job believing in us. Now you just must believe in yourself. From now on, in everything you do, make sure you do it with full confidence in yourself, your abilities, and your good feelings. You just believe, and the rest will come by itself.

Well, you can now open your eyes a little at a time and stretch your whole body carefully. We have successfully completed this session. I congratulate you for your great work. Rest and see you next time.

The Person You Will Become

Greetings! How are you feeling this time? I hope you are doing great and enjoying unparalleled physical and mental health. Health is the most important thing, and, therefore, it is the most wonderful thing we can wish for another person.

I am very happy to be here with you once again in this new guided meditation. The following experience is something a little different from the others, but do not worry, just because it is different does not mean you should be afraid of it. Just relax and enjoy.

Previously, we traveled to the past to correct our traumas, or we brought our attention to the present moment to calm our thinking. Well, this time, we will take a small glimpse into the future. More specifically your future, and the kind of person you want to become someday.

One of the many keys to achieving success and accomplishing your goals is visualization. So, let us visualise the kind of person you would like to be in about 5 years. Who would you feel? What would you wear? What would you like to do for a living? What would your attitude towards life's problems be like? Whatever those answers are, we will find out next.

Always remember to be very honest with yourself. You do not have to keep anything to yourself or meet anyone's expectations, just being you is enough.

Do not be nervous, remember that I will always be here to go with you. I am your friend, and I will take you by the hand throughout this experience, so just let yourself go. Are you ready? Perfect then, let us get started.

Start by finding a comfortable place where you can begin to meditate. This can be your room or someone else's, a study, a beautiful garden, or terrace, or even a park full of nature. Make sure that there are no disturbing noises and that no one will disturb you while you meditate. I will give you a few moments to find your ideal space. I will be right back; take your time.

Once we have our ideal meditation space, we will proceed to sit on a comfortable and peaceful surface. This can be a chair, a sofa, or an armchair; even your bed is good for this purpose. I will give you a few moments to choose.

Okay, now let us check that posture. The recommended posture is with your back always straight but without exerting tension on it. You can place a cushion behind your back if you feel uncomfortable, which in turn will correct that misaligned posture that you always carry in the day.

Let your arms fall, and your hands rest on your lap, relax your legs and let your feet rest comfortably on the floor. Relax your abdominal and back area, let your shoulders, neck, and head fall under their own weight, and release all tension from your facial muscles. Let go of all accumulated tension; we do not need it.

That is it; I see with joy that you have finally achieved a proper meditation posture. I congratulate you. Proceed to close your eyes little by little and begin to breathe using your diaphragm. Breathe in a slow and very deep way, bringing all your attention to your precious breath. You know how it is, so let us proceed.

Inhale, inhale at this moment, fill your abdomen as much as you can with oxygen... and now exhale, releasing all the tensions contained in your body together with the warm air coming out of your mouth. Remember to give yourself a short pause at the end of each breath. Good, you are doing great. Our body breathes at its own rhythm, and we simply focus on how it does it.

By focusing on our breathing, there is no more room in our minds to concentrate on our fears or any other negative thoughts. A focused mind does not get carried away by negativity.

Continue to breathe, do this until you become fully aware of your breath. I will leave you alone for a few minutes so you can concentrate as much as you can. I will be right back.

Okay, that is it. You and your breath have become one once again. Congratulations. Now, we will focus on a little exercise but continue breathing as you have been doing so far. It is time to start with the visualization; imagine the person you want to be and how you will feel in the future. Think that all the lessons you have learned here have led you to the success you so desired.

What do you see? Is that you? Dig a little deeper and try to feel the emotions of that future you. How do you feel right now? There is a warmth in your chest like you have never felt before in your life. Now we know that smile is not fake; it is a sincere reflection of the well-being you have achieved in the future.

Achieving love, reaching your dreams, your goals, none of these things seem impossible at all. You may not be able to see the future in its entirety, but you do know one thing. You will become happy, fulfilled, wise, and very confident. You left behind all the negativity in your life to become the person you always wanted to be inside.

Congratulations, you have officially made it, and if you believe in yourself, you will make it in the future. Be thankful because everything you have visualized is already yours. That is true.

Well, now you can open your eyes and stretch your body little by little. We have finished with this session. See you, take a rest.

A Better Version of Yourself

Hey there! I bet all this was a gigantic journey of self-discovery for you, wasn't it? Do not be afraid, it was for me too, and truth be told, I am very glad I went through it with you.

We learned several tools along the way to help you heal and be the best version of yourself. We learned to calm down and breathe, examine our bodies for impurities, connect and take pride in our inner selves, and constantly remind ourselves how beautiful, amazing, and wonderful we are; we even learned how to use quantum physics to heal our own cells. That is completely crazy stuff, don't you think? But it was all real, wonderfully real.

Still, I want you to always keep something in mind, something you should never forget. The human brain learns by repetition; there is no other way. If we tell ourselves one hundred times that we are beautiful, we will be right, and if we tell ourselves another one hundred times that we are not worthy, we will also be right. Therefore, it is better to repeat positive things until we believe them, and they come true.

Where do I want to go with all this? You may ask yourself, although I think at this point you already know the answer to this, my friend. It is not enough to just apply what you have learned for today or tomorrow; it is not even enough to repeat it for a whole week, a month, or a year.

If you really want to see a change and become that happy person you are so eager to become in the future, you will have to incorporate all these healthy habits into your day-to-day life.

The key to consistency and adaptability. Start by making small changes in your daily routine, say nice things to yourself in the mirror, congratulate yourself for a job well done, pamper yourself, and occasionally give yourself a well-deserved treat.

Remember, you deserve to be treated the same way you treat other people. If you treat others so well, why not do the same to yourself? You deserve a lot of good things too.

Just do not incorporate all these changes at once, or you run the risk that the corrupted file in your mind will reject them and continue to infest your mind. Think of it like starting a new diet, you cannot replace all those foods you like all at once, or you will be more likely to give in to temptation and abandon the diet in a heartbeat.

Ironically, that is something that happens all too often. When people do not see quick results, they end up giving up on their goal and go back to the old corrupt, negative program.

So, what to do? You may ask. Well, this is where consistency and adaptability take place.   As I said, start by making small positive changes in your life, be consistent, and little by little the old program will be replaced by the newer, brighter version.

We cannot expect to change a negative mentality that has been brewing for years in our minds in a matter of a few days. It does not work that way. If we want to see significant changes, we will have to start reprogramming ourselves day by day.

I know it may sound complicated, but in truth, it is as simple as adopting a good habit. If day after day you wake up, look at yourself in the mirror and repeat to yourself with a lot of encouragement that you are a winner, then eventually your brain will start to believe it. If you keep it up for a while, guess what will happen? Exactly, your subconscious will transform you into the definition of a winner that you have in your mind.

Have you ever heard that we make our reality ourselves? Well, let me tell you that there is no truer truth in the history of mankind. Think of it this way, the brain learns and interprets everything it sees throughout life; therefore, if you experienced something traumatic, your mind would begin to interpret the events of your life concerning that trauma.

Experience shapes our thinking, and our thinking shapes our whole life. That is why visualisations and meditations play an essential role in overcoming any traumatic event. On this journey, you free yourself from everything that hinders your growth. So, go ahead and change once and for all, implement these meditations and positive exercises in your daily life.

Do not be afraid, you can do it. You can move forward and overcome all trials. Remember that you can use your creativity to solve problems and set new goals to keep yourself alive. Surround yourself with positive people; use humor to take the weight off difficult situations; listen to these guided meditations to relax and increase your concentration; and find creative tasks, such as painting, singing, or doing something that makes you feel good.

After all, the first step to being a winner is to believe that you are already a winner. I believe in you; now, you just need to do the same. Every time you feel doubts, remember that inside you have all the tools you need to move forward, and every day you are getting closer to being the best version of yourself!

As a gift to you, I have added a free bonus workbook that you can work through to help you understand where your negative thoughts and feelings come from and how you can change these. Complete each exercise from the workbook buy drawing your own ginger bread person and following the directions on each worksheet.

I sincerely hope you have enjoyed this book and use the scripts as many times as you consider to help you reprogram your negative thinking and elevate your energy to a state of peace and healing. Thank you for allowing me to accompany you on this journey. Namaste!

"Make today the first day of your preferred life"

THE BRAIN AS A SUPERCOMPUTER AND HOW IT AFFECTS OUR PHYSICAL AND EMOTIONAL WELLBEING

Quantum physics and mind and body, how negative and positive feelings can affect our mindset. Free Bonus printable workbook

Workbook

MARIA SAYER

THERAPEUTIC COUNSELLOR

How we think and feel can affect our physical health and mental health

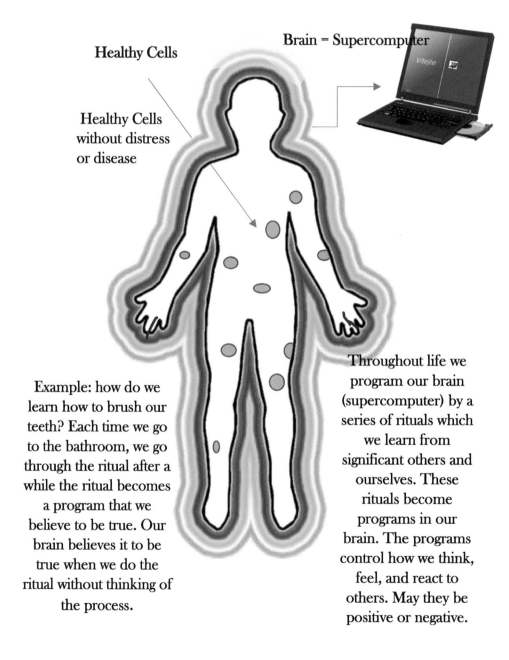

Healthy Cells

Brain = Supercomputer

Healthy Cells without distress or disease

Example: how do we learn how to brush our teeth? Each time we go to the bathroom, we go through the ritual after a while the ritual becomes a program that we believe to be true. Our brain believes it to be true when we do the ritual without thinking of the process.

Throughout life we program our brain (supercomputer) by a series of rituals which we learn from significant others and ourselves. These rituals become programs in our brain. The programs control how we think, feel, and react to others. May they be positive or negative.

Did you know if you have enough trauma in your life, whether it is physical trauma, emotional trauma including stress & anxiety? We can alter our cells in our body, which in turn can rewire our supercomputer so that we become more negative and always expect the worst in life, together with this we can cause our healthy cells to become in distress. Which then can turn in to disease.

When I say disease or distress, we alter the structure of our cells this can make them unhealthy which you may then experience things like IBS, Migraines, Cold Sores, Coughs, and colds etc. Theorists know this may happen, and as a result you can either rewire your body/brain to expect the worst / catastrophise.

If we can alter healthy cells to become distressed, we then can alter change distressed cells to become healthy through positive rituals and self-talk.

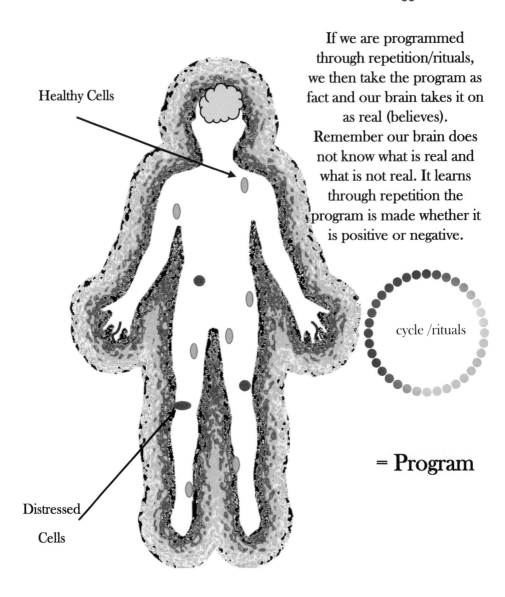

If we are programmed through repetition/rituals, we then take the program as fact and our brain takes it on as real (believes). Remember our brain does not know what is real and what is not real. It learns through repetition the program is made whether it is positive or negative.

Healthy Cells

cycle /rituals

= Program

Distressed Cells

This is then where we make our mindset, if we have a lot of negative in our lives, we then wire our brain to expect the worst – so this is where the saying comes in "you get what you speak."

We have the power to change this, but we often struggle as to how?

If the negative gets put in our minds and body through repetition before we take it on as fact, surely, we then can do the same using positive talk and rituals?

Negative, thoughts, experiences, and feelings I have/had

Sit in a quiet place and complete the following exercise.

On the next page there is an exercise that may help you to see and reflect on all the negative experiences, people and things that have been said to you over the years. Be honest and write everything down.

Once you have written everything down, draw a line through everything that **DID NOT** come from you originally. I am aware that this may be a significant percentage of what you have written.

Questions to ask yourself:

- Did you have control over the situation? If no cross it out!
- Did you wake up in the morning and say I want to feel this way if no cross it out!
- Do the feelings from this belong to you, or are they from something else? If something or someone else "cross off"
- Are the feelings a result of something that you had no control over? If yes, cross it out!

Repeating this process will enable you to identify what is your stuff and what has come from external events, people, or situations that you do not have control over.

Remember yes, you did feel these feelings at the time, but... do you want them to continue to hurt you in the present and future? If no, let them GO! They serve no purpose only to remind you that you have been hurt.

Remember, most of these feelings you hold are from things, people, or events that you had no control over.

We have a choice as to whether we hold on to the feelings and let them continue to hurt us or, We can deconstruct them, see who they belong to and choose to discard and replace by positive feelings.

So, you ask yourself if this can be done?

Well, we can! I am not saying it is easy, but it is achievable by reprograming and changing the corrupt files in our brain that have been placed there usually by others through repetition until our brain believes them and they become a program.

Let us start to deconstruct our negative feelings on the next page.

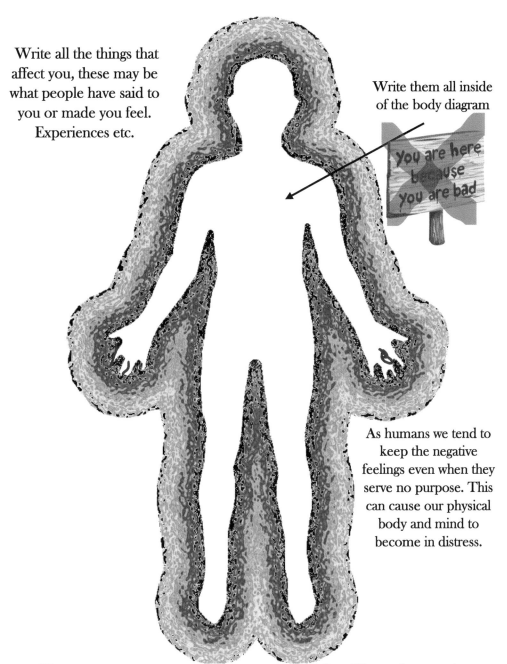

Write all the things that affect you, these may be what people have said to you or made you feel. Experiences etc.

Write them all inside of the body diagram

you are here because you are bad

As humans we tend to keep the negative feelings even when they serve no purpose. This can cause our physical body and mind to become in distress.

Turn over to next page to see an example of how devastating negative words can have on a person, how they program and believe it to be true and how it affects all their life (ripple effect)

An example of negative program and how it may affect a person?

Repetative

You are Stupid!
You are Stupid!
You are Stupid!
You are Stupid!
You are Stupid!

RESULT

I AM STUPID!

RIPPLE EFFECT

How it affects everything we say or do?

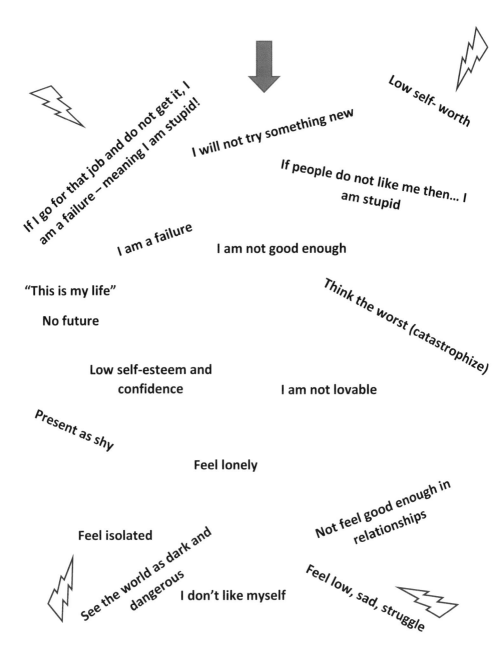

Low self- worth

If I go for that job and do not get it, I am a failure – meaning I am stupid!

I will not try something new

If people do not like me then... I am stupid

I am a failure

I am not good enough

"This is my life"

No future

Think the worst (catastrophize)

Low self-esteem and confidence

I am not lovable

Present as shy

Feel lonely

Feel isolated

Not feel good enough in relationships

See the world as dark and dangerous

I don't like myself

Feel low, sad, struggle

We could go on and make these more personal to each person

The Preferred Self – Who I want to be

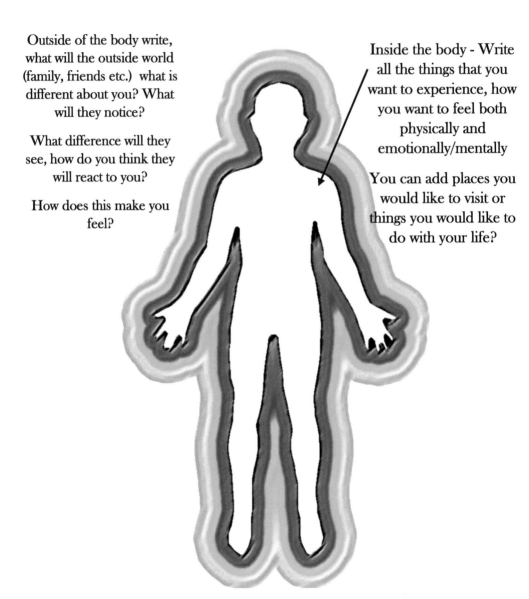

Outside of the body write, what will the outside world (family, friends etc.) what is different about you? What will they notice?

What difference will they see, how do you think they will react to you?

How does this make you feel?

Inside the body - Write all the things that you want to experience, how you want to feel both physically and emotionally/mentally

You can add places you would like to visit or things you would like to do with your life?

So, what is stopping you from achieving this? Turn to the next page to find out...

So, what is stopping you from achieving this?

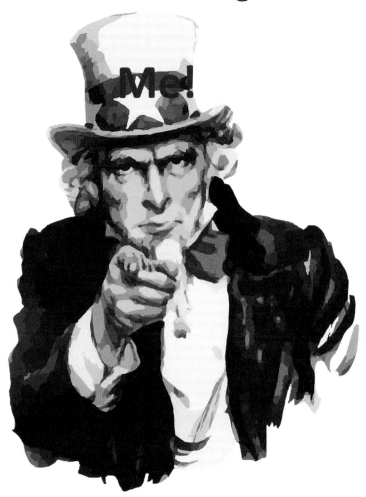

This is how we change our mindset
and heal our distressed Cells

**Start today, to have the life
you want, not what you
expect...**

Little steps

Repetitive (repeatedly)

Reprogram

Change your mindset

Result - happier/healthier outlook on life (Positive outlook)

How we can change our mindset and heal our distressed Cells in our body

Write down all the things you will do to change your negative mindset to a positive one. Remember we do this through repetitiveness (the same way the negative was programmed into us) This is the way our supercomputer brain gets programmed.

Here are examples of affirmations, make your own or use these.

- I am fantastic
- I choose to be happy
- In life I will get speed bumps, I will not allow them to negatively affect my present and future.
- I am beautiful
- I am clever
- I am good enough
- I am lovable

- I can do this!
- I am a Winner

What is your favourite colour? Wear it often to remind you. Say the colour in your mind, this equals being positive

What things make you smile?

Tai chi

Yoga

Exercise

Do something new? E.g., hobby, try new foods, music etc.

Smile – release dopamine!

Pay it forward – do not expect anything back. Enjoy making someone else's day.

Focus on doing the things that make you feel happy, content, grateful, etc. let go of the things you have no control over as these are the things that distress our brain and body

When you are thinking about how you will change your mindset, break it down into small steps. E.g., if part of your plan is to travel and you do not have the means to do it yet. Learn the language of the country where you want to go to. Check out their customs and traditions. Have a themed night at home eating foods from that country, listening to their music etc. Visualise yourself there feeling content and enjoying every moment of it.

Our brain does not know what is real and what is not real, through repetition it learns programs. Programs become facts this is when the brain believes them as true. Which means this is when you believe them to be true.

Remember every little step together with other positive steps makes a program in your supercomputer.

Use the worksheet on the next page to plan

From today I will...

Remember be specific, break it down for example:

If you want to feel happy, what would that look like, how would this make a difference to you? What would you be doing?

I want to feel proud - break it down, what would this look like, what would you be proud of?

My message to you

"Throughout life we will experience what I call speed bumps (negative experiences, feelings and people)

We can...

Chose to let the negative experiences etc. affect us

Or

We can choose to deflect them back to where they have come from.

We do not have to take on other people's/

experiences/words and feelings.

We can choose to be happy

Or

We can choose to be sad.

However, the more you learn to deflect other people's negative thoughts and feelings the more you can be that healthier and happier person. Which will allow you to deal with 'speed bumps' better in life"

"Let us get real, do you want to
continue to bare the effects of
other people's rubbish they
have bestowed on you?
Or
Do you want to be the decision
maker in your life as to how
you want to feel and be?"

M Sayer

In memory of Mary Margaret

McClymont

Printed in Great Britain
by Amazon